WHAT IS ACUPUNCTURE?
HOW DOES IT WORK?

WHAT IS ACUPUNCTURE? HOW DOES IT WORK?

by

Dr. ERIC H.W. STIEFVATER

With Three Appendices by the Translator,

LESLIE O. KORTH, D.O., M.R.O.

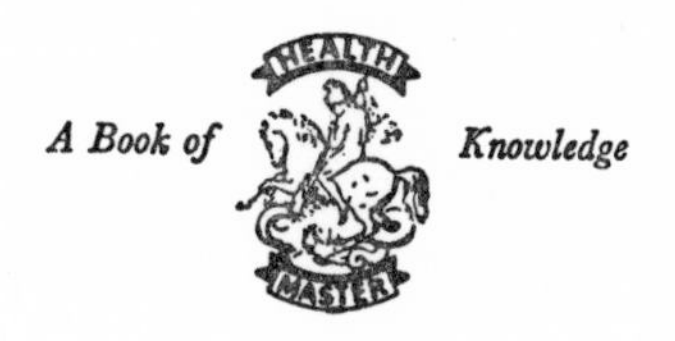

HEALTH SCIENCE PRESS

BRADFORD, HOLSWORTHY

DEVON, EX22 7AP, ENGLAND

First Edition (translated from the German) 1962
Second Edition (revised, enlarged and reset) September 1971
Second Impression April 1973

ISBN 0 85032 087 9

Typeset in Great Britiain by Specialised Offset Services Ltd., Liverpool
and printed by Weatherby Woolnough Ltd., Sanders Road, Wellingborough.

CONTENTS

FOREWORD

This short introduction to acupuncture is intended to awaken interest and to invite further study. It will be readily appreciated that the whole extent of the problem of 'Oriental Medicine' cannot be dealt with in only a few pages. In this regard we are not yet scientifically or perhaps humanly sufficiently prepared in spite of the many publications.

I should like to emphasise that the works on acupuncture – and also the work here – must certainly be differentiated from the popular European style of Eastern philosophy. Furthermore, acupuncture should not be used (by confused minds) as a secret path to a medical religion. Here it is a matter of the practical application and clear understanding of a healing method, not of speculation not of mystery. To be sure there is an element of primordial medicine in acupuncture. But of reform no one should speak who does not recognise the great value of reform and the shortcomings of one's own ability.

I have written this brief work for two reasons: firstly because, as already stated, I wish to further the general interest in acupuncture: then secondly because I believe that our so very standardized medicine should also opportunely get to know other presentations and methods. Undoubtedly it is very uncomfortable to tear oneself away from the accustomed trains of thought; but intellectual discomfort can prove profitable and is necessary.

Finally, may this publication also correct those false and exaggerated presentations, which have arisen through many sensational reports. Acupuncture is neither a 'cure-all' nor a historical curiosity. It is a possibility among other possibilities to aid the sick. It is a good foundation-stone – for the *building up of an individual healing art.*

Erich W. Stiefvater

FREIBERG i.Br. October, 1955

THE 'ART OF ACUPUNCTURE'

Whoever, for the first time, sees an antique picture of acupuncture is purplexed by the complicacy of the lines and points which are recorded on the framework of a primitive human body. The first impression is one of confused pedantry. Involuntarily a comparison with the classical Chinese opera forces itself upon one, in which the head posture, the position of the feet are laid down precisely, even up to the movement of the fingers and the direction of the glance. But not only by observing the pictures, but also by reading the old texts the kindly disposed adepts of Eastern healing-wisdom would easily have been discouraged had they not repeatedly found points which revealed just as great a wisdom as a close observation of nature. These encourage them to delve deeper into the remarkable 'system of acupuncture'. Gradually the dry material becomes vivified. After years of patient work the ancient ways of expression become understandable; one learns to distinguish between the eternal truth and the current false. After further patient *accomplished practice* one enters still deeper into the wisdom of this healing art.

Acupuncture in Europe

Acupuncture has not been known all that long in Europe. Only in 1683 there appeared a joint publication by a Jesuit missionary and a doctor of the East India Company on the Chinese pulse and acupuncture. It belongs, even today, to the most thorough and sensible works on acupuncture. But only at the beginning of this century did a few European doctors commence seriously to occupy themselves with acupuncture. However, as was to be expected, it remained at the few. For all that, during the last few years interest seems to have spread.

Two Essential Qualities

Acupuncture is a difficult healing art to learn. To state it more precisely: it is learnable only up to a certain point. The greater part depends upon the innate ability of the doctor and on the sensitivity of his touch. These two qualities are a gift of the gods like the gift of music or sculpture. But even the godly endowment is of little account if its possessor does not develop it through practice.

WHAT IS ACUPUNCTURE?

The unsophisticated reader of the word acupuncture has at once the unpleasant feeling of a *needle* and of a *prick*. Now it is like this: the acupuncteur introduces very fine, special needles into the skin at quite definite points. As a result of a special technique (practice!) this needle-prick is only a trifle painful. Again and again are patients surprised that the needles have already been introduced; they had imagined it to be much worse. But, as a matter of fact, the needles are not the deciding factor, but the precise area of their application. It is on the knowledge and discovery of over 800 points on the body surface that the greater part of the art of acupuncture rests. This statement should have a quietening effect upon the reader. He will at once see that this treatment requires a meticulous examination of the skin. Acupuncture trains the doctor in an extraordinary, practical – indeed in a fine, artistic cultivation of his hands. In this lies hidden the genuine wisdom of the East. He who would comprehensively grasp this should read that *wonderful* book by Eugen Herrigel, *Zen in der Kunst des Bogenschiessens* (obtainable now in English as *Zen in the Art of Archery*): likewise that enlightening work by Graf Dürckheim: *Japan, oder die Kultur der Stille (Japan or the Culture of the Silence).*

But we are only at the very beginning of our investigation of acupuncture. On closer study one stumbles upon one surprise after another. This very ancient form of medicine looks upon many things in man more in a primordial sort of way. Our customary medical technical formulae sometimes bar the way to the primordial. In many respects we must alter our way of thinking; not that we must disregard our modern achievements, but that we comprehend the primordial more accurately.

THE CHINESE PULSE THEORY

Let us at once begin with one of the most difficult chapters, i.e., with the system of the so-called '14 Chinese radial pulses.' Even today this widespread form of diagnosis in the whole of the orient is mysterious. We are unable to grasp it according to our present day physiological ideas. It demands a very delicate sense of touch in the fingers. For this reason it is very subjective and is, therefore, rightly considered to be scientifically untenable. *But it exists.* The phenomenon of the Chinese pulse diagnosis has two important marks of distinction, namely, it is very ancient and is used over an extensive geographical compass.

How to Feel the Pulses

The 14 Chinese pulses – as is the pulse with us – are felt on both radial arteries; not with one finger, but with three fingers next to each other *and* at the same time in two or three different pressure strengths. Thus the state of six different organs is to be ascertained under the three fingers on the radial pulse.

Now it must be mentioned that even in ancient China this form of diagnosis was not the only one. The Chinese physician employed a differential observation of the countenance, its expression, its colour and especially of the eyes. He questioned his patient very thoroughly. He used a specialized abdominal diagnosis; the abdomen, it is stated, is the 'Centre of Energy.' Likewise no modern doctor would exclusively employ the Chinese pulse diagnosis. He would rather bring it into the framework of his other (and customary) diagnostic methods of examination.

Quintessence of Pulse Diagnosis

Sometimes, however, it can be that this pulse diagnosis draws our attention to organs which we, with our modern methods, do not recognize as being affected. Now we may criticize this pulse diagnosis as we will, it must, at all events, give us cause to think that it applies to an extremely delicate reacting system, namely, the circulatory system which is animated, rhythmical, uninterrupted, efficacious. For the rest one finds, from the 'scientific standpoint' much that is laughable; but when one is hard pressed one often seizes – from deep instinct – upon the laughable. In this respect life offers sufficient examples. The quintessence of the Chinese pulse diagnosis is this: it endeavours to establish from the strength and form of the pulse under each palpating finger, whether the corresponding organ is underfunctioning or overfunctioning. To know this is surely of great significance for quite a number of therapeutic applications.

ON THE SO-CALLED 'PERIPHERAL PULSE'

Acupuncture knows of yet a second, let us say complementary method of pulse diagnosis. This I should like to designate as the 'peripheral pulse'. In China it is called 'revealing pulse'. Each organ possesses such a one. This pulse I consider to be of extraordinary significance. It is situated at various points of the body where the arteries run relatively near to the surface and are, therefore, palpable, such as on the head, neck, arms and hands, also below the inguinal fold, in the popliteal space and feet. It is obvious that these blood vessels have a definite anatomical and well-known connection with the internal organs. If one compares the results of examination of the 14 radial pulses with those of the peripheral, then one often finds a conformity or very striking supplementations.

The examination of the 'peripheral pulse' leads to the examination of many points on the body surface. I have already hinted that I look upon this examination as, so to speak, the 'All Highest' of acupuncture. Here is a field for steadfast practice; here the opportunity to penetrate the secret, wonderfully significant content of every single small region of the body with its inner relationships. But for a complete mastery of this art a knowledge of the rules is necessary – and this theoretical knowledge of acupuncture is very difficult to acquire (because so difficult to grasp).

THE 'YIN' AND THE 'YANG'

Ancient China thought somewhat differently about the processes of the human body, about health and disease than does modern, scientific medicine. Man existed completely in the rhythm of the moving life surrounding him. Reducing it to a single formula one might say: the Chinese viewed man as being ruled by those *two great forces,* which govern also our earth and our heaven. These forces they named the 'Yin' and the 'Yang'. Yin signifies dark, cold, moist proceeding from without inwardly to the centre.

Yang is in contrast thereto: light, warmth, dryness radiating from the centre outwards. These two forces are active also in man. *When they are in equilibrium,* man is healthy; but if one over-balances one or the other too much then 'disease' arises.

THE THERAPEUTIC POINTS OF ATTACK

Now the therapeutic attack – the healing art of the Chinese – consists in the restoration of harmony of both of these fundamental forces, *or to prevent the disharmony taking place in the first instance.* Thus acupuncture is really a very old and very important *form of hygiene.* And in this sense it is only logical that the Chinese physician was paid for the healthy days of his patients and not for the sick ones.

THE PRACTICAL WAY

To maintain this balance and to restore it in the case of illness is a great art. Let us start with an example. When someone today suffers from sleeplessness he can compel sleep by taking tablets. Everybody knows that such a 'treatment' is powerless to remove the disturbance of the equilibrium which causes the sleeplessness. The real basis of the disturbance is not done away with. One may well imagine that the inner disquietude caused by the inability to sleep can be taken as nature's warning of a developing hidden disease. This can lie in the physical or in the mental spheres respectively. We do not strike a child when it cries because it is hungry;

but we stifle, without question, the call of the body for help. The body speaks its own silent yet clear language for those who have ears to hear and eyes to see. Sleeplessness is one of those ever recurring messages from the animated body, as for example is also pain (and pain in a certain area!) or fatigue, as well as disturbances of elimination, lack of appetite, skin colour and many other things. But let us return to our subject. How then will acupuncture remove the disturbance of the equilibrium in a practical way? In this respect a discussion of a few fundamentals is essential.

AN INGENIOUS DISCOVERY

There are Yin and Yang Organs

One of the most ingenious conceptions of the Chinese medicine is the division of the principal organs of the human body into a Yin character and a Yang character. No one knows how, in the course of history, this came about. Today these things are reported in the available textbooks on acupuncture as a matter of course. Yet they should be thought about very deeply, otherwise no conclusion will be arrived at. Surely the Chinese have anticipated something, what we today have recognized as 'SYNERGISMUS', the harmonious play between the *vagus and sympathetic* within the *vegetative nerve system.*

Hollow Organs Subject to Yang

It is of extreme significance that the hollow organs

are subjected to the energy form of Yang; one could also say that they are the organic representation of this principle. As hollow organs the Chinese recognize: stomach, small intestine, large intestine, gall bladder. The hollow organs are of movement (peristaltic), active, eliminating (centrifugal).

Dense Organs Subject to Yin

The dense organs are under the influence of the energy of Yin, i.e., they are massive 'sluggish', 'dark'. The dense organs are: liver, kidneys, heart, spleen, pancreas, lungs. Now we already know that the adjustment of the balance of energy in the body amounts to how much the activity of the hollow and dense organs are in harmony with each other.

Heart and Vessels as Yin-organs

The Chinese also knew of the regulation of warmth and appropriately attributed it to the force of Yang. On the other hand they ascribed the Yin principle to the heart, the blood vessels and the glands of internal secretion, in so far as these were known to them. We are accustomed to look upon the heart and vessels as hollow organs; but in acupuncture they are considered as being co-ordinated with the blood, and therefore, as is the blood itself, are treated as Yin-organs. Blood is mass. It does not move of itself; but is moved. By what? We say today: by the heart and by the blood vessel system. And what power moves the heart? That we do not know, because we do not know what Life is and what is the life-force. Most probably '*Life*' is not at all knowable.

THE 'CHINESE MONAD'

This system might have something about it that is boring for the layman, and something quaint and unproven for the doctor. But, as already stated, with patient deliberation this system will be found to be based upon 'intelligence' which each organ has within itself. Let us try to make this clear by an example. The liver is considered to be a 'dense' organ and therefore as a 'YIN' organ. It is a quiet, massive organ of a dark colour; it contains much fluid, but it is not absolutely a Yin-organ for although quiescent, a secret life is active in it. That is the 'small Yang', that is buried in the 'large Yin' of the liver. So there is in each Yin-organ a little Yang, and in each Yang-organ a little Yin. This, Chinese wisdom has represented in the symbol of the 'Chinese Monad' thus:

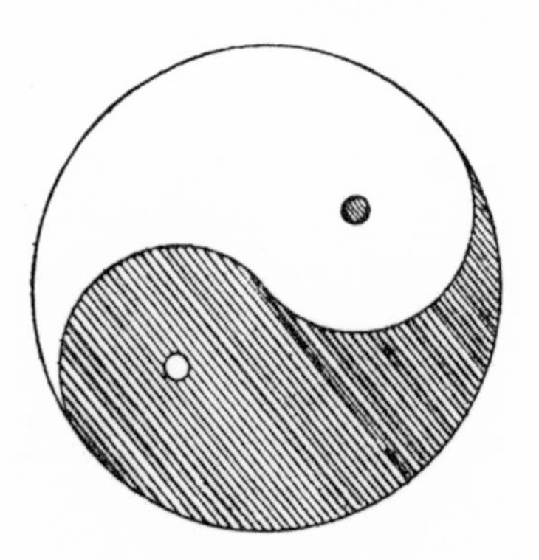

One could easily look upon this symbol as a pictorial form of Einstein's theory of relativity.

Mutual Dependence of Mind and Body

Still more surprised are we to learn that the liver – that large subterranean factory – is styled 'the seat of the Unconscious.' Why should there not be something of a truth in this? We are aware that damage to the functioning of the liver can cause a 'gloomy' mood and a disposition to worry and grief. Conversely anxiety, sorrow and anger can damage the liver (also the gall bladder). It has not yet been sufficiently ascertained in how far 'swallowed anger' is responsible for the formation of gall stones. The most sagacious statement on these questions was recorded by Paracelsus in his book on *The Tartaric Diseases.* It must once again be stressed that the investigation of the Unconscious should be devoted to organic functioning rather than to mythology in relation thereto. Man is a body with a soul and not a dictionary. Thus, in many cases, the purport *'of psychical states is inferred from damaged organs,'* as, conversely, is an organic failure due to a kind of psychical handicap. How very much are body and mind dependent upon each other! The 'purport' appears to be both mental and physical. It appears to be the one as well as the other. It must be more primordial, ancient, than the conscious act of thinking, which can say to itself: I am worried, I feel pleasure, I am excited. It must be something living, something like a memory of a condition in which we are unable to think that the body and mind *could* be separated.

A SECOND INGENIOUS DISCOVERY

Thus the Chinese knew that one could not treat an organ without, at the same time, touching the mind. But here at this point, we become acquainted with a second ingenious discovery of Chinese medicine. One *observed* that the *expression* of 'internal' diseases appeared on the surface of the body, namely, on the skin and through the skin. *The discovery of the relationship of internal organs (and thereby also the mind) to the skin is the result of brilliant observation of nature, and is one of the greatest accomplishments of Chinese medicine.* There really must have been many thousands of Chinese doctors who, over many centuries, have studied man with unending patience before this system could have been developed that we describe as the 'system of the 14 meridians of acupuncture.'

Meridians are Real Though Invisible

These *meridians* are thought out, they are invisible, but nevertheless 'paths', actual tracks, over which the organs report changes in them from the depths of the body to the surface. We can now well understand also that these meridians, corresponding to 'their organs', are divided into Yin and Yang-meridians. Even today we can easily imagine how the discovery of these paths came about. It must have been just the same in the primitive beginnings of acupuncture as it is today when 'it' pains us anywhere for we 'involuntarily' grasp, press and massage those parts. Later one noted certain ever recurring painful spots and, at the same time, observed their connection, by lines, with the organs suspected as diseased. Finally it did not require the specialized medical technique of the twentieth century in order to *see* that in heart disease there occurred blue lips, an altered pulse rate, oedema of the feet and sensations of pain on the inner side of both arms; or that in gall bladder complaints pain in the right hyper-gastric region, in the feet and hip-joints and symptoms over the right eye could be found. All these symptoms were observed in ancient times, in part better than in the present day, when a certain craze for measuring with apparatus dulls the vision in regard to the simple phenomena of life. The diseases of mankind have always been basically the same; only their designations and manner of their treatment have changed. (*See Appendix One*).

Now the ancient acupuncture, that seemed so confusing at the beginning, has surely become somewhat clearer to us. Anyway, we are now acquainted with the fundamentals. The knowledge of its particular technique and refinements, the relationships of meridians and points one with the other and their combinations represent the long road that the practitioner of acupuncture must travel if he will progress from knowledge to accomplishment, from apprentice to master.

DIFFERENT FORMS OF ACUPUNCTURE

As already mentioned at the outset, in the classical form of acupuncture fine needles (silver, gold, also steel) are introduced into definite points of the skin. One often hears from European doctors that this is nothing special. Such a tiny needle prick is insignificant practically. The modern doctor gives injections daily, whereby it does not depend upon the needle, but, in the first place, on the medicament used.

Significance of the Body Surface

Certainly the present day injections are made in virtue of the medicament itself. No significance whatever is attributed to the prick or prick-point. Usually injections are given in two ways: intravenous in the vein of the arm, and intra-muscular in the muscle of the buttock. Every layman knows this nowadays. Of the many sided phenomena, which, however, a single prick along brings about in the body, modern medicine has made but very little observation. The attention of modern medicine rivets itself far too much on medicaments. That has its reasons, also its blessings.

Medicaments have been at all times an important part of medicine But it was given to the Chinese to recognize also the significance of the body surface for a therapy having manifold stimuli, in conjunction with a wealth of medical remedies. They not only introduced needles into the skin, but they burnt so-called 'moxas' on certain areas of the skin. (*See Appendix Three*). Furthermore they had a unique form of massage.

Acupuncture Without Needles

Through the intelligent use and improvement of massage, and through the discovery of the 'segments' of the skin (segment therapy) we have today a much greater understanding of the possibilities of acupuncture than in former times.

This segment therapy consists of making small weals on a definite skin area by the injection of a certain drug, sometimes only of air. This is nothing but unconscious acupuncture. One recognized then that not only the medicament, but also the spot in which the injection was made was of significance. So it was a matter of the much quoted 'catch-word': 'the know-how'!

I personally value the *acupuncture without needles* just as much as with, because I hold the view that there is no better remedy, no more delicate an instrument, no better blessed healing means than the *hands of the doctor.* This *'acupuncture with the hand'* consists of a special meridian massage and point massage, by which one, without doubt, can exercise a direct influence upon the internal organs. It requires a delicate touch, years of practice and great patience on the part of the doctor as well as on the part of the patient.

It is interesting to read that in the latter period of mesmerism the magnetic stroking movements (the so-called 'passes') were carried out by direct contact with the skin, i.e., it became a kind of massage. The paths along which the hands travelled correspond, in many respects, to the acupuncture meridians. One sees that the *fundamentals of the therapy,* as of diseases, are always the same; only the names change in accordance with the conception, which we have of disease at the time.

ACUPUNCTURE AND HOMOEOPATHY

It is therefore obvious that such a system should be combined with modern therapeutic technique. And why not? It is not a matter of cultivating acupuncture as, so to speak, an antique show piece. We are not living in the China of the middle ages or before the birth of Christ. If acupuncture has in it a genuine, valuable and vital quality then it will be adaptable to any period of time and can be beneficially combined with any sensible medicament, any valuable technique. We have only then really inherited an ancient good thing, when we developed it on up-to-date lines. Life is development, change. The Chinese philosophy of medicine teaches, more than anything else, the idea of constant change. The new becomes old, the old becomes new. A fine example of this is afforded by an occurrence in the history of homoeopathy. Round about 1880 a homoeopathic doctor by the name of *Weihe* observed that in certain diseases certain points on the skin became painful. These areas on the skin he named after the specific remedy that was indicated for the particular disease and spoke, for example, of a lachesis point, digitalis point or graphite point.

The French physician and acupuncteur Dr. de la Fuye also observed this when he undertook to compare the Weihe points with those of acupuncture. He found that a certain number of these points coincided exactly with each other. Thus did de la Fuye come to combine acupuncture with homoeopathy. He named the system '*homoeosiniatrie.*'

Relationship Between Acupuncture and Homoeopathy

The proper and true relationship between acupuncture and homoepathy has, however, a deeper basis than that of the Weihe points. First of all: both curative systems have originated quite independently of each other. But both include the great significance of the symptoms of the sick. These symptoms are the language of the animated body, of our human nature. One should not underestimate them (certainly they should not be overestimated either). Modern medicine prefers chemico-physical methods of examination. It questions the body about details – and it does not always understand these aright; for it is the body's way to answer in complex pictures, not in isolated ones. A tree brings forth apples, but not so many units of weight of fruit sugar, fruit juices, cellulose, vitamins. Rather are apples natural entities. We are able to analyse but never to synthesize them. We must not appraise the physico-chemical answers of the body too little, but never too much either. When the human organism says: my blood pressure is too high, then this is manifested in the symptoms in the occurrence of headaches, giddiness, ear noises, visual disturbances, weakness of the intellect. It cannot say: I have a blood pressure reading of 250/150. This we arrive at by measurement. The physician must pay attention to both together, namely, the figure and symptoms.

The first point of agreement between acupuncture and homoeopathy lies in the consideration of the symptoms. A second point we find in the therapy: *both systems work with small stimuli.* These work slowly and are far-reaching; they influence the constitution; they are harmless and are quite in accordance with the processes of nature.

For these two reasons homoeopathy and acupuncture supplement each other beautifully. The art of a combined homoeo-cutaneous therapy consists in evolving a suitable remedy in accordance with the symptoms, *and at the same time* giving the appropriate skin treatment to the disturbed area of pent-up energy.

A PRACTICAL EXAMPLE

Numerous individuals suffer from *disturbances of the portal circulation* due to their sedentary way of life. Continual sitting posture, usually in a vitiated atmosphere, reduces respiratory movements of the chest and diaphragm. The 'sitter' breathes *shallowly.* As an added misfortune he smokes frequently. So an impoverishment of oxygen of the body is brought about: *desoxybiose.* We must therefore lift a warning finger: badly aerated cells are in danger of cancer. When the diaphragm scarcely moves, the normal respiratory massage of the liver is practically nil. In consequence of insufficient movement of the legs, and, over and above this, the squeezing of the hip and knee-joints (and thereby of the adjacent blood vessels) *congestion of the lower extremities* takes place. The consequences, observed from above downwards, are: damage to the liver cells, digestive disturbances (above all, constipation), haemorrhoids, varicose veins, oedema, cold legs and feet, leg ulcers. This symptom-complex, occurring in many modifications, can, for example, be beneficially influenced homoeopathically with remedies for the connective tissue, blood vessels and liver. Results, however, occur more quickly when one, at the same time, treats according to the principles of acupuncture, those points, which have a special relationship to the portal vascular system and to the liver itself.

The Chinese would say: here the principle 'Yin' preponderates (the Yin-organs, whose meridians have a particular relationship to the legs, are: liver, kidneys, spleen and pancreas). These points are situated, in part, over those important blood vessels and nerve paths for the blood supply and movement of the legs but they are also significant for the blood supply of the liver, spleen and kidneys. One could almost say that a few of the points exercise a *sluice function.* (In ancient Chinese schools of medicine the circulation of the blood was demonstrated to the students as a highly artistic pump and pipe system). Simple pricks, massage or small injections on these points could change the disease-picture for the better in a short time. A thorough improvement in unfavourable working and living conditions rounds off the treatment.

'HARMONIZING' THE NERVOUS SYSTEM

Many doctors will not like this word at all. I should like to explain how I came upon it. From what has already been said emerges how very appropriate a thoroughly understood and, at the same time, modern acupuncture is as a basic therapy, or as a supplementary treatment. It has been proved in practical work that acupuncture is able to alter the reactivity of the body. We know how very often tried remedies have not had any effect. Obviously the nervous system of such individuals is in a state of lessened reactivity. By applying delicate stimuli to this nerve system a sort of sensitization can be achieved, and thereby a better response to the medicament.

To use a simple example: the best artist cannot produce good music if the strings of his instrument are not correctly tuned. This the acupuncture treatment of the human body attempts to do: it purports 'correctly' to harmonize the nerve system. This, however, can only be possible by application of minute stimuli.

ACUPUNCTURE AND SEGMENT THERAPY

The greatest interest in acupuncture up to now, is to be found in that branch of medicine, which is styled 'reflex-zone-therapy.' This form of therapy is based on the discovery – involving the nerve structure – that there are certain areas (segments) on the skin which, as a *field of expression of the internal organs,* are most impressive. Thus there are segments of the heart, liver, kidneys, intestines, stomach, etc. These segments become hypersensitive very soon after the onset of an internal disease and painful later on. This sort of diagnosis is for the not yet 'objectivized' early stages of disease, of very great importance.

Acupuncture amplifies and extends this modern reflex zone treatment by virtue of its ancient experiences, its highly differentiated knowledge of the surface of the human body and by its revolutionary conception of what modern medicine calls 'reflex'.

Let us learn to understand this concept somewhat better.

THE 'CIRCULATION OF ENERGY'

Old ideas can become revolutionary when the time is ripe. In quite a general way one can say: the body reflects every stimulus. Observing a single stimulus we are able to speak of a single reflex. But during the course of life we have to do with unceasing, changing stimuli. We are always subjected to repeated, unending, finely graduated consequences by manifold stimuli of food, weather, light, psychical impressions. All this takes place in a kind of circulatory manner from morning to night, from spring to autumn, from youth to old age. These stimuli come about in the form of repeated cycles. Is it then so wrong-headed to think also that the energy of our body-mind, which is continually being awakened by these stimuli, moves itself in a circulatory kind of way?

The classical example, or better stated: the prototype of all circular forms of movement in the body is the circulation of the blood. But we should not consider it too isolated. Could it not be also that the tissues and organs nourished by the blood and the processes taking place within them proceed in daily and seasonal cycles? The Chinese might have thought in this way when they formulated the third ingenious idea of their medicine, namely, that the organs of our body have, in the periodic cycle of a day-night-entity, quite definite times of rest (accumulation-phase) and of work (elimination-phase). The ingenuity of this line of thought does not rest on its speculative beauty, but on its being won by the observation of man.

THE CHINESE ORGAN CLOCK

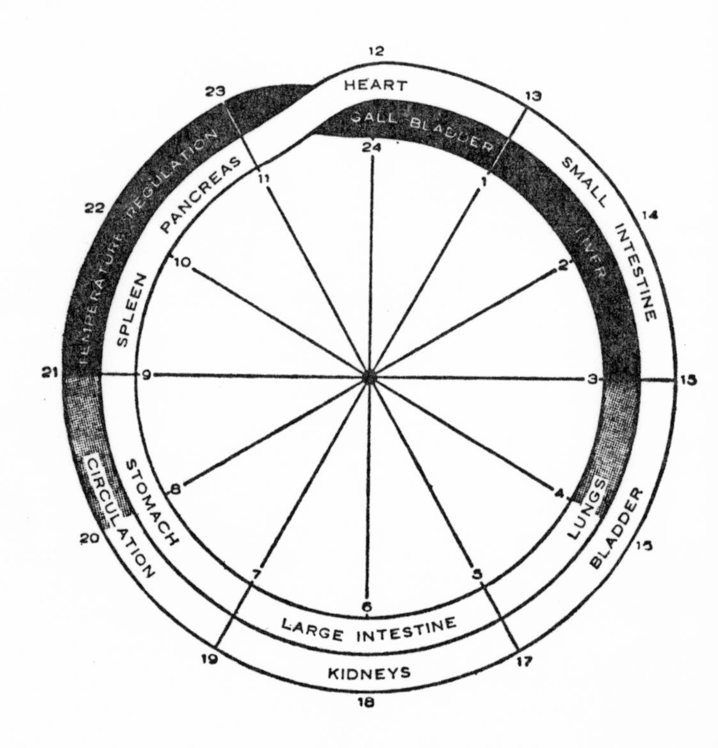

The Chinese constructed a twenty-four-hour clock from which could be read the period of rest and of activity of the twelve organs of the body. They expressed it thus: energy circulated through an organ every two hours. On the other hand, it is a puzzle how they were able, with their simple means of observation, to allocate to each organ the 'correct' two hours. These were named the 'organ maximum times' (OMT). See this clock in the facing illustration.

A Valuable Diagnostic Aid

When we see, for example, that the large intestine has its organ maximum time in the morning from 5-7 o'clock, then we can easily recognize the reason for this classification, namely, at this time the large intestine is in its main emptying phase. From this we can already draw a therapeutical conclusion that between 5 and 7 in the morning the large intestine reacts particularly quickly to 'purgative' treatment. We can now apply such a consideration to every organ. Many times we shall be able to confirm the correctness of the Chinese organ clock out of our own experience. Modern research in rhythm has worked out an appreciable number of exact measurements on organ rhythm, which coincide with the Chinese observations to a great extent. When we compare all these observations without prejudice and check up on them ourselves by practical application, then we have in our hands a very valuable new diagnostic means. In this means lies the possibility of assessing symptoms, occurring at a certain hour, as relating to a specific organ. When, for example, a patient states he wakes up nearly every night between

1 and 3 o'clock, then that is a pointer to a disturbed function of the liver. We should then subject this organ to a closer examination.

More especially valuable is the organ clock for the *timely classification of pain.* We are aware of the great importance, for example, homoeopathy attributes to the many kinds of pain. Now here we have the possibility to draw a conclusion from the particular hour of occurrence of a pain in the organ that has caused it. Every layman knows that gall bladder colic usually takes place at night time. Now the organ maximum time for the gall bladder is actually at 11-1 o'clock at night.

Timing for Administration of Remedies

The acupuncture therapist can not only draw certain diagnostic conclusions from the organ clock, but he has in this a good indicator for the time of administration of correct remedies (especially homoeopathic). When the organ clock is divided into day and night halves, then we are able to associate the function of assimilation with the night half and elimination with the day half. To know this is certainly very important for the administration of remedies that induce elimination and promote nutrition and building up.

Crisis Periods

Furthermore the doctor must keep his eye particularly on the 'transitional hours' at which the change from the day half to the night-half takes place. These transitional hours are crisis periods. It is an old medical experience that at 3 a.m. most cases of death occur, because of the low blood pressure and of the reduced heart function. We also know that after the midday meal, from 1 to 3 o'clock a phase of fatigue sets in. At this time the individual is usually unable to accomplish much. One should draw conclusions from this fact.

Everyone, so to speak, carries within himself his own 'inner clock'. I believe, from what has been said, that it is important to get to know this clock and to heed its warning.

As with everything else that human nature forces into a definite scheme, so also will the organ clock have its shortcomings. If, however, we look upon it as a practical help, as a method, as a working hypothesis, then we shall use it rightly. We progress over our mistakes only through practice in the avoidance of them.

THE FIELD OF APPLICATION OF ACUPUNCTURE

It is really not quite correct when anyone asks about the 'field of application of acupuncture', i.e., about the diseases, designated by modern names, which can be 'cured' by acupuncture. A question put in this way misses the real purport of acupuncture. We have seen that the whole idea of acupuncture lies in the influencing of the mind-body reactions. The whole purport of acupuncture is to get behind the disease. There are so many conditions which we call disease. We will not, in the first instance, treat each disease separately but effect a *bodily adjustment to them.*

Acupuncture for Everyday Troubles

Experience teaches that this is best done at the commencement of a disease. The Chinese state in their very ancient book of wisdom *I Ching:* one can change things so long as they are in being. Hence acupuncture attends to early diagnosis and early treatment. Only secondarily is the 'matured' disease considered. To the former belong all those forms of illness which we style as 'functional,' i.e., with few tissue changes and accompanying disturbances. To treat a perforated appendix or an infarcted heart with acupuncture would be a gross professional error. But the many cases and forms of skin disorders, neuralgias and rheumatic complaints, migraine, asthma, functional disturbances of the bladder and kidneys, gall bladder affections, functional disturbances of the stomach and intestines offer a wide field for acupuncture. These numerous 'everyday' troubles are, in contrast to the severe organic complaints necessitating clinical treatment, by far in the majority. They determine our daily condition, our ability to do things. They are also the precursors of worse things, warning signs of coming afflictions, and this we must never forget.

Here is the field for acupuncture; here is its justification.

A FEW CONCLUDING THOUGHTS

The treatment with acupuncture presupposes a certain calmness and poise. It is not just a matter of dealing with palpation of the body surfaces, of feeling the pulse, of the interrogation of the patient, of the introduction of the needles or the carrying out of special massage in the turmoil of daily life. This treatment is no 'magic' as one embarrassed critic would have it, but a challenge to one's conscientiousness and humanity. There are methods of treatment which one can neither describe as individual nor as corresponding to the dignity of man. The acupuncture treatment distinguishes itself by an intensive search into the whole nature of the patient. One must say that there is no pain, no feeling so trifling that it must not be considered by the doctor. The human organism has sometimes a loud, sometimes also a gentle, practically helpless voice.

Let us remind ourselves once more, that the Chinese understand by 'energy' something universal, almost God-like. The work on this energy in man, i.e., on his life energy, and the insight into its mysterious intermingling with the organs, with the mind and with Time must give us over and over again a feeling of wonder and awe.

APPENDIX ONE

THE MERIDIANS

The Chinese acupuncturists claim that there are fourteen meridians in the body which transmit a current of energy feeding the main organs, i.e., stomach, heart, lungs, kidneys, and so on. Too strong a flow or a too weak one along the course of a meridian can result in a disordered function of the respective organ, leading to an illness. The disturbed flow can be restored by stimulation through the pricking with the needles on the specific points of the meridian, of which, so it is asserted, there are approximately 800.

Some Western medical doctors have shown scepticism about the meridians, but it has been found possible to trace them by the use of an apparatus which indicates that their paths evidence less resistance to electricity than other parts of the skin's surface. Furthermore the pricking of some of the 800 points along the paths under treatment does change the electrical condition.

A Japanese doctor has invented a unit which records the beats of the fourteen pulses. This appears to lend support to the Chinese theories that meridians do exist and that stimulating them at the specific points changes their state.

The pain of angina pectoris, a mystery still to the Western medical profession, usually runs from the heart down the left arm to the little finger, which is exactly the line of the Chinese heart meridian.

A theory advanced by a professor at the Gorki University is that the acupuncture needles that are inserted into the nerve endings convey electrical impulses along the nerve fibres to the spinal cord, then to the lower centres of the brain and from there back to the various organs of the body: a reflex action.

APPENDIX TWO

THE PRESSURE METHOD OF ACUPUNCTURE

1. FINGER PRESSURE

The finger is to be pressed firmly on the area that is found to be tender. In the treatment of some diseases this method is found to be effective.

It is simpler than the needle pricks or moxibustion, and can be used with advantage on children and on those adults who also have an aversion to the needle pricks. The same sensation can be obtained on several points with finger pressure, as with either the pricks or moxibustion. This applies particularly to tender points in the region of the temples, ear, the face, the shoulders, the upper chest, and also to points on the extremities.

The pressure can be exercised with the finger-nail or with the finger-pad of one, two or three fingers, namely: the thumb, forefinger and middle finger, depending upon the thickness of the muscle layer.

This method has, in general, many advantages and is easy to carry out. It is recommended for pain, first and second degree burns, and insect bites. In these cases the finger pressure is to be made somewhat distal to the painful spots. The pain usually ceases on pressure. It is possible for the pain to be dispersed or even hindered from developing.

2. PRESSURE WITH A METAL ROD

A rod with a pear-shaped head is used nowadays, but in ancient times a thin rod with a rounded head and a thicker one with a ball-shaped head were in use. The thin rod was used on patients who feared the pricks of the needles, whilst the ball-shaped head was employed for massage.

The thin rod, or the modern pear-shaped head, can be used as a substitute for the finger pressure, especially on points where finger pressure is difficult to apply.

In the treatment of muscle pains of rheumatic origin a rocking movement should be made with the fingers in all directions on the same spot. Massage can be carried out also on the adjacent points.

The number of treatments depends upon the nature of the complaint and varies considerably with the patient.

We must bear in mind that in the Far East

acupuncture, in the main, is a preventive method. In Japan, before the occident invasion, about 1860, everyone was under the obligation once in every three months to be treated by acupuncture or moxa. In this way the patient under examination was, in the majority of cases, not ill, the needling being employed when the special radial pulses (Chinese Pulses) indicated some disturbance of the balance of energies. In such a case a single treatment every two months sufficed to maintain health.

Unfortunately it is different in Europe, when the doctor is consulted only in the event of illness.

As already stated, the number of treatments depends mainly upon the nature of the disease, the individual manner of reaction and the constitution of the patient.

APPENDIX THREE

MOXIBUSTION

Moxa or moxibustion serves a similar purpose to that of acupuncture, i.e., to bring into proper balance the flow of Yin and Yang.

As Dr. Nakayama has stated: moxibustion, called also ignipuncture, is based on heat. It is therefore of the nature of YANG. Consequently it is directly indicated in all diseases that are caused by the excess of YIN.

The practice of mixibustion consists of the application to the skin of combustible cones made from powdered leaves of *artemisia vulgaris.* These cones are ignited and placed on particular spots. They are extinguished only after they have burned down to the skin and (in some cases) allowed to form a blister.

Moxa can also be applied to the acupuncture points **AFTER** the needle has been withdrawn.

Some **MODERN** Japanese physicians have studied moxa and acupuncture by means of modern laboratory methods in order to determine whether the treatment really activates the inherent curative powers beyond just having a psychological effect.

Dr. Nakayma, the outstanding scientist in this group, has collected the conclusions of some of his colleagues. For example, one of the scientists, Dr. Hara, after long studies pursued over many years, has not so long ago made available laboratory proofs that demonstrate that moxibustion actually increases the number of red blood corpuscles and haemoglobin. The needles have a similar effect.

Dr. Nakayma's own conclusions were reached after the completion of a great number of clinical tests which showed that a vast variety of diseases had greatly improved after application of either moxa or acupuncture. The doctor found that both these therapies exerted a great influence upon the blood itself, a fact that seems unbelievable. It is true, however, that not much improvement or difference is noted immediately after the first treatment. But through controlled moxibustion carried out for some length of time, the blood is found to undergo a striking and important transformation. Experience also teaches that the needles produce even quicker results. Dr. Nakayama stated further that since moxibustion represents a physical therapy of the nature of **YANG**, it should be used to cure all excess of **YIN**.

But moxibustion, being in fact a physical stimulus, also animates all physiological functions in a general way. It aids metabolism; it activates the leucocytes and the nervous and psychic centres. In so far as physico-pharmaceutical stimulus is concerned it also exercises an equally favourable and efficacious influence in troubles having the nature of Yang.

Dr. Nakayama's statement reflects the point of view and methodology of a **MODERN** physician having a firm belief in the validity of the system of Yin and Yang.

It is astonishing to see that moxa, which is one of the oldest remedies in existence and mentioned in the most ancient Chinese medical treatise, was used in Hiroshima on August 6th 1945, and actually brought relief to one of the sufferers from the effects of radiation from the first atom bomb. Mr. John Hersey in his book *Hiroshima* tells that twenty-five to thirty days after the explosion, blood disorders appeared; gums bled, the white-blood-cell count dropped sharply. The two key symptoms, on which doctors came to base their diagnosis, were fever and the lowered white-corpuscle count.

One of the survivors, the Reverend Tanimoto, who was a graduate in theology and who was two miles away from the centre at the time of the explosion, fell ill about two weeks later with general malaise, weariness and feverishness. Since his health did not improve he sought medical help. He was given injections of vitamin B_1 but these did little to improve his condition. After a few days, however, a Buddist priest, with whom Mr. Tanimoto happened to be acquainted, called on him and suggested that moxibustion might afford relief; the priest showed the pastor how to give himself the ancient Japanese treatment by igniting a twist of the stimulant herb and where to place it on the wrist. Mr. Tanimoto found that each moxa treatment temporarily reduced his fever by one degree. Dr. Nakayama's research on the effect of moxa upon the blood makes one appreciate the instinctive wisdom of applying moxibustion in this case. It can be safely assumed that had the treatment been continued for an extended period, it might have caused a quicker recovery than was achieved by the methods used. But even the temporary relief effected by this ancient form of therapy is surely an indication of its great value, which found its first expression in the Yellow Emperor's Canon of internal medicine.

Moxibustion is a kind of cauterization, which reaches back in its history to the mists of antiquity. There have been very many means of bringing about this cauterization, but here we are dealing with moxibustion.

Small plugs or cones are made from flax fibres,

chiefly of a certain kind of yarrow or tansy. Moxas are also made from the pith of sunflowers, lint, cotton wool, fungi. These cones are ignited and after slow burning they leave behind a small scar about the size of a pea, and according to numerous reports by travellers from the East, this treatment is most effective, astonishingly so, even in cases of trigeminal neuralgia, sciatica, neuritis, arthritis and rheumatism, etc.

The localization of these artificially induced burns, many of which are made at the same time, is determined by experience, which has proved itself over a long period of time and in a similar manner as the *Feu Chirugie* (Fire Surgery) or *'Point de Feu'* (Point of Fire) of the Arabs and Hindus. The localization of areas corresponds frequently to the reflex zones or pain zones of Head.

The determination of points, diagnosis and methods of application are largely the same as those of acupuncture. If it is a case of skin disease, moxibustion may be applied in accordance with the size of the affected part. In cauterizing with moxa-rolls care should be taken to see that the skin of the patient is not burned. The distance between the glowing end of the 'moxa-cigarette' and the skin should be such that the patient can only feel a comfortable warmth. Generally speaking the time required for moxibustion at each point should be from twenty to thirty minutes, but it may vary according to circumstances.

Some practitioners recommend impregnation with

saltpetre, but others object to this because the burning must not take place too quickly.

The part of the body to be treated must be protected by a damp cloth, in which a small opening is made to admit the moxa. The moxa cone is then lighted at the top. Some press the moxa on the skin with tweezers until it is completely burnt. If necessary the glow is maintained by blowing.

The patient feels pain only from the lower end, which can be pretty severe at first; but then it quickly subsides, and according to the strength of the treatment so will the degree of the resulting scab be, over which a salve is to be smeared. This is to be kept on for eight to ten days, when the scab falls off.

Treatment, however, can be made on the Chinese acupuncture points on the same principle as moxa, but without its troublesome application and painful effect of the ignited cones: in France today certain practitioners employ a small thermometer-like tube in order to bring about the heating of the skin. The small tube is filled with hot water and applied to the part five to seven times at short intervals. According to the reactivity of the patient's skin, a more or less distinct blister is formed: its reabsorption acts as an auto-vaccine.

I myself find that an improved kind of moxa treatment can be achieved by the use of cupping glasses. A small ball of cotton wool is soaked in methylated spirit, held in a pair of tweezers, ignited and placed on the painful area, then speedily covered over with the cupping glass. The flame not only creates heat but also a vacuum in the glass by burning up the air in it. The vacuum causes the encompassing flesh to be sucked up into the glass, thus producing a strong hyperaemia on the surface that relieves deep congestion and accelerates the circulation.

In my book *Some Unusual Healing Methods* I have devoted a chapter to the technique and usefulness of the cupping therapy, which is extensively used in France (Ventouse) in Germany (Schroepfen) and elsewhere on the Continent. It is an uncomplicated, but most effective remedial agent. Indeed the effect of the ordinary orthodox moxa treatment can be greatly enhanced by following it up with therapeutic cupping.

Moxa therapy is especially renowned in the East for its cures of many complaints such as paralyses, serious discharges, *tumour albus* (white swelling), T.B., meningitis, gout.

In Japan moxibustion is used in **CHRONIC** cases and the needles in **ACUTE** ones, but according to Nakayama preference has been given, since ancient times, to moxa in the treatment of disease, and today we are beginning to understand how compression massage works in the light of the Chinese and Japanese systems of healing.

HOW TO USE MOXA ACCORDING TO ANCIENT TEACHING

Question: How do you use moxa to effect a burn and how much moxa is required?

Answer: You make a very small wad out of wool between the fingers, not larger than a pea. The upper part is pointed, the under part flat. You place the under surface on the spot where the burn is to take place. You ignite the pointed end with a fusee, which gives off a pleasant odour.

Q. Does the woollen-like material ignite easily?

A. If it is thoroughly dry it ignites very easily.

Q. Will the wad burn completely to ashes?

A. Not quite. There will always remain a little of the wad which does not become ash.

Q. How is it that the wad is not completely consumed by the flame?

A. By the moisture, that is absorbed from the affected part by the burning wool, going mostly up in vapour; some of it remains in the burning wad and damps it, so that it cannot burn wholly to ash.

Q. Do not these scorchings create small blisters on the skin?

A. Not at all. They cause small grey patches, even after the ignited wads have been applied several times consecutively on the same place.

Q. What explanation can be given that no blisters are caused by the flame?

A. None, other than that the small wad does not burn right down to the skin, it being only marked.

Q. Does not the marking cause severe pain?

A. The pain is tolerable owing to the material being of a light consistency and not firm or thick; furthermore the wad is small and does not burn down to the skin.

Q. Does the burning of the wad last long?

A. Not longer than one can count up to fifty.

Q. How often does one apply the burning wad on one spot?

A. Generally three times on a weak tender skin, but oftener on other parts as may be necessary until the complaint has gone. For example: in the case of hip-pain up to twenty-five wads, indeed up to fifty on the same place, from which one need not fear the slightest harm, but rather a definite relief can be expected.

Q. But does not the marking cause any after-pain?

A. None at all. With the extinguishing of the flame the treated part can be directly touched without any appreciable discomfort being experienced, indeed even if the spot be prodded or pressed.

Q. Does the marking completely drive out the pain wherever it may be in the body, or only lessens it?

A. Both: even up to the verge of the miraculous.